A Way With Pain

D0716590

A LION BOOK

Oxford · Batavia · Sydney

Text copyright © 1990 Mary Batchelor
This edition copyright © 1990 Lion Publishing

Published by
Lion Publishing plc
Sandy Lane West, Littlemore, Oxford, England
ISBN 0 7459 1600 7
Lion Publishing Corporation
1705 Hubbard Avenue, Batavia, Illinois 60510, USA
ISBN 0 7459 1600 7
Albatross Books Pty Ltd
PO Box 320, Sutherland, NSW 2232, Australia
ISBN 0 7324 0169 0

First edition 1990
All rights reserved

Acknowledgments
All photographs, including cover, supplied by Zefa (UK) Ltd

British Library Cataloguing in Publication Data

Batchelor, Mary
  A way with pain.
  1. Man. Pain. Toleration
  I. Title
  152.1′824
  ISBN 0 7459 1600 7

Library of Congress Cataloging-in-Publication Data

Batchelor, Mary.
  A way with pain / Mary Batchelor. — 1st ed.
  p. cm.
  ISBN 0 7459 1600 7
  1. Pain—Popular works.   I. Title.
  RB127.B37   1990
  616′.0472—dc20

Printed and bound in Yugoslavia

CONTENTS

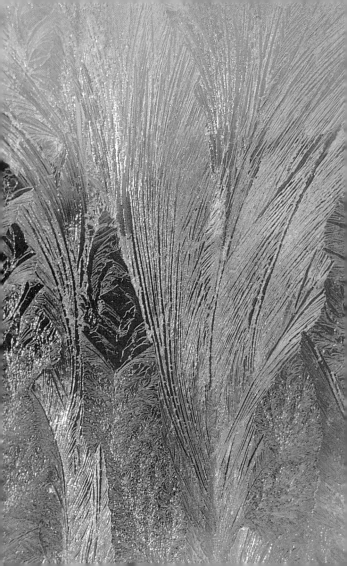

1

For People in Pain

We have all had our share of pain — starting from the time we cut our first teeth.

But for some — those with chronic pain — it is an unwelcome ingredient of everyday life.

Chronic pain is pain that lasts longer than a few months, that occurs often or continually and that fails to respond to treatment. This book is written for all who are trying to learn to live with it.

I am trying to do so myself. Since my teens I have suffered from various forms of arthritis. In spite of the best endeavours of doctors, I have to live with pain.

To find out more about the subject, I consulted doctors, psychologists, and others who treat pain. I read books on the subject. Above all, I talked and listened to others with chronic pain of one kind or another.

I learned a lot, and I hope that the insights, information and practical tips I gained will help some of the other people who face each day — and night — with the handicap of pain.

A handicap can *be overcome. Sometimes it may even be turned to advantage. Once we have some understanding of the problem, and of ourselves, we shall be better equipped to do so.*

With courage, and God's help, we can live successfully with pain.

2

Different Kinds of Pain

Chronic pain is pain that has come to stay. There are various causes of such pain. The most common are:

- arthritis — which involves disease or damage to the joints
- rheumatism — a general term that covers aches in the bones, muscles, joints and tissues surrounding the joints
- lower back pain
- neuralgia — sometimes following shingles
- pelvic pain, in women
- generalized abdominal pain
- pain from adhesions, following surgery, or scars that pull
- pain following injury after accident, especially where the weight-bearing limbs are affected (e.g. legs).

Doctors distinguish between organic and functional pain. Organic pain can be diagnosed from

X-rays or other tests. When pain is functional, it is just as real, but the doctor cannot discover the cause. Lower back pain, pelvic pain and generalized abdominal pain may fall into this category.

Those suffering from functional pain often feel especially vulnerable.

It is accepted that stress and anxiety can cause physical pain, but that does not mean that the pain is all in the mind. In time, tests may be devised which indicate organic causes, or new causes for non-specific pain may be discovered.

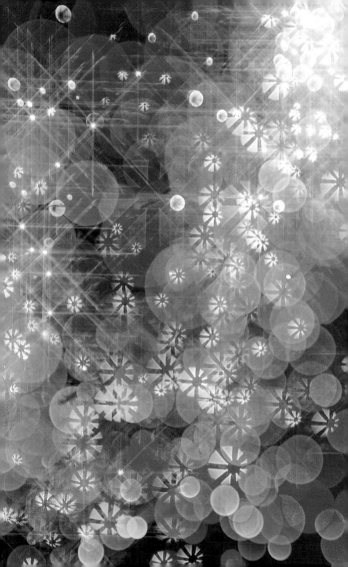

3

Why? — And Why Me?

Some people have been saddled with ill-health from birth or childhood. Others are left with pain as a result of illness or accident, disease, or deterioration of joints and muscles.

Both groups are likely to ask the questions, 'Why?' and 'Why me?'

It is natural to want to make sense of our lives. We feel better able to come to terms with our situation if we can understand the reason behind it.

'It was the job in the factory, handling chemicals.'

'It was because I had four pregnancies so quickly.'

'I think I inherited it from my mother.'

'I've never been the same since an injection I had in hospital.'

'It's my temperament — I worry too much.'

'I must have done something to deserve it.'

'It was the drunken driver who caused the accident.'

Some lay the blame at someone else's door. Others blame themselves, and add guilt to their load.

Maybe I can't track down a reason for my pain. That does not mean that I cannot make sense of my situation. I need to find meaning in the *whole* of life — the good bits as well as the bad.

Those who believe in God — the loving, caring, all-powerful God of the Bible — find it easier to believe that there is a pattern in everything that happens, whether or not it is obvious at the time. That belief helps them to handle their pain.

When God is in control of my life he can help me to discover something positive in everything that happens to me — including pain.

But then if God is good, why does he let us suffer? The problem of pain in the light of a good and loving God is one of life's biggest mysteries. The Bible tells us that suffering is *not* God's choice for us. If our world was run on God's lines, there would be no pain.

But from the beginning, men and women chose to disobey God's laws and guidelines and go their own way. Just as breaking ecological laws has brought terrible consequences, so breaking God's laws has resulted in pain and suffering that affect innocent and guilty alike.

Pain has become part of the human lot. That being so, we might as well ask, 'Why *not* me?' as question why we should be picked on to suffer.

The good news is that God has not washed

his hands of our world, or left us to sweat it out alone. In the person of Jesus, he became one of us and experienced pain himself. He knows all about suffering at first hand, and is willing to be with us in it, sharing our pain.

4

What is Pain?

We all know what pain feels like, but what exactly is it?

We feel pain when nerves near the injured part carry messages to the brain. So pain is physiological.

But, as one doctor explained: 'There are many components to pain. There is the actual nerve damage and the message carried up your nerve to your brain. You have to have an intact nervous system to feel the pain at all. But you also have to have a brain that tells you something about what you are feeling. And that is coloured by a hundred and one other things.'

Some people feel pain more — or less — than others. Everyone's pain threshold is different.

We would all like to be able to calculate the level of pain we feel. But a doctor told me: 'Pain is always subjective. There is no way of measuring it. My patients tell me what *kind* of pain they have — colicky, sharp, throbbing or dull — but not how intense it is. I can only guess that from how severe the patient perceives it to be.'

A professor at a London hospital writes:

'The simplest of pain is never simple. An apparently straightforward pain in my leg or my stomach may be produced by a whole network of causes. Anxiety, fear, hopelessness, anger, sleeplessness and inactivity all play their part.'

The complex character of pain helps to explain why it is sometimes worse — or better.

It means that if I sort out some of the hidden emotions and come to terms with unresolved areas in my life I am likely to make the pain easier too.

5

Is the Pain Real?

**I want the doctor to stop my pain, but I also want
to be told that the pain is real.**

**If doctors tell me to stop worrying, or to
live a less stressful life, are they saying that if I
stop worrying, or change my lifestyle, the pain will
disappear?**

There's a mixture of reasons for most pain we
experience. We can't isolate our bodies from the rest
of us. What happens to my body is coloured by
what is going on in the rest of me. All this, in turn,
is influenced by my circumstances and relationships.
Every part of my life affects every other part.

When Jesus was on earth, he cured physical
illness. But more than that, he offered wholeness.
When a paralyzed man was brought to him, he dealt
first with the man's broken relationship with God.
He told him that his sins were forgiven. Afterwards
he cured his paralysis.

Today, as then, those who reach out to Jesus for
help, find wholeness of a new kind. The physical

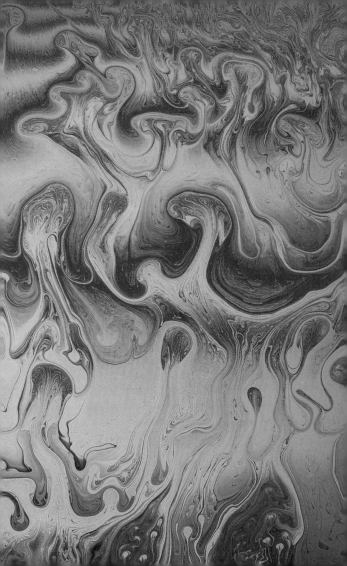

cause of their pain may not disappear, but the
forgiveness and new life which he gives will have its
own beneficial effect on mind and body too.

Some approaches to pain are not honest or helpful.
According to one theory, if I tell myself often
enough that I have no pain, it will disappear. That
just is not true. It is not 'positive thinking'
to pretend that the pain does not exist. I must
recognize that it is real if I am to find ways of
dealing with it.

Others say that it does not matter whether the
pain is real or imagined. They see no need to
distinguish between organic pain and pain which
results from non-physical causes.

But those of us at the receiving end of treatment
must try to disentangle the different strands that
make up the pain. Then we can set about finding
ways to relieve it.

6

Can I Find Healing?

When we first go to the doctor in pain, we are likely to be sent for X-rays and tests, in order to determine the cause. Hospital tests, and the treatment that may follow, help us to feel that something is being done. The problem comes later, when everything has been tried, and nothing has stopped the pain.

Some of the trouble may be our own fault. We may have too much faith in medical science and expect cures where none have yet been found.

When medicine fails to help, some people wonder if God will work a miracle and heal them, like Jesus did when he was on earth.

Some people today *do* experience miraculous healing. But for every one who does, there are many others who come to God with equal trust but receive no physical healing in answer to their prayer.

If we are to make sense of this seeming inconsistency, there are a number of key points we must hold on to:

- *All healing comes from God.* The body's natural healing process — whether we cut a finger or break a bone — is part of God's design, and a miracle in its own right.

- *Doctors and medical personnel are agents of God's healing.* So are those who research new ways to heal and relieve pain.

- *God is not ours to command.* He does not respond automatically to our requests, like a heavenly vending-machine.

The Bible talks about the 'fear of the Lord'. This does not mean that we should be frightened of God, but it does remind us that he is far greater than we are and has knowledge and plans beyond our understanding. We need to recognize and respect this truth about God.

God has the right to choose when and how he will heal. He can be trusted to know what is genuinely best for us, even when he allows pain and disability to continue.

- *Healing is much more than freedom from pain and disease of the body.* When we ask God to heal, he does so at a profound spiritual and emotional level, even when the physical pain remains.

- *God can help us to accept our pain without bitterness.*

- *God can show us how to live lives full of meaning and purpose in the midst of pain.*

- *God can show us positive ways through the situation.*

● *God can give us strength to bear our pain.*

Some Christians say that if we ask with enough faith, God is bound to heal our bodies. But this conclusion is false as well as cruel. God deals with us as individuals. He does not answer all prayers in the same way.

All pain ends at death — but death is not the end of life. The kind of life that God offers to us now, through Jesus Christ, survives death. It begins in the present, but it will be enjoyed fully and completely when we 'go home' to be with God, where there is no more pain.

7

Whose Life is it Anyway?

'I really don't think the doctor can be bothered any more,' Sue complained.

To be fair, the doctor had done her best and tried all kinds of treatment.

When no more can be done, it is hard for both the doctor and the patient. We should not let the relationship become soured at this point by our persistent visits and demands for help.

When orthodox medicine fails, many people go from one qualified — or unqualified — person to another, looking for help. It is reasonable to explore alternative treatments, but spending our lives chasing a cure does more harm than good. It concentrates our attention on the pain and puts off the time when we come to terms with our situation.

Eventually I must take responsibility for myself and my pain.

Janet put it this way: 'Ultimately, I am alone with my pain. That means that if I don't take care of myself, no one else will. Doctors are not likely to remain interested or make rules for me when they can't relieve the pain any more. It's up to me to plan and organize my life so as to cope in the best possible way.'

Janet lives alone. But even when we are part of a family unit, we should not let someone else take over responsibility. We need to make our own decisions and plan how best to use the energy and abilities we still have.

8

Challenging the Limits

**When we allow pain to narrow our horizons
and limit our range of activities, we create more
and more no-go areas for ourselves. So a decision,
instead, to 'opt in' and take responsibility for
ourselves and for the control of our pain, may
involve changes in lifestyle.**

There is growing recognition that exercise helps to
relieve pain. Many people rest painful limbs or joints
to avoid pain, but lack of use causes muscles to
waste and makes the pain worse. Centres and groups
are being set up to teach people to begin using
muscles and joints that have been out of action for
many years.

*Peggy, who is is sixty-five, has suffered from curvature of the spine since she was fourteen. Her lower back
muscles have become almost rigid. Now, at a hospital
day class, she is practising push-ups, with a target of
twenty a day.*

Walking is one of the best forms of exercise. We

can all help ourselves by increasing, little by little, the distance we walk each day.

Doing things we enjoy is good therapy too. An adviser at a hospital unit asks her patients what they would most like to do, if they were not disabled and in pain. She helps them get as near as possible to reaching that goal, whether it is to go swimming again, or to get to the local library on their own.

We can all set ourselves targets, and aim to take up hobbies and interests that will give enjoyment and a sense of personal achievement as well as doing us good physically.

Sometimes fear makes us narrow our horizons — and not just fear of the pain. We may be afraid of not being able to cope as well as others who are completely fit. When we have not done anything for a long time we lose confidence. This can apply to going out of the house on our own, travelling by train, driving the car, or accepting an invitation to dinner.

If we are to broaden our horizons we need courage to overcome the butterflies in the stomach, as well as the physical pain. We shall need patience. We can increase the range of what is possible only by easy stages. But, little by little, we can push out the boundaries and begin to open doors instead of closing them.

9

Practical Hints

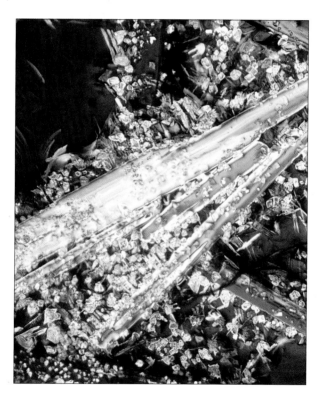

We may look wistfully at advertisements for wonder cures but, deep down, we know that we must be realistic about our pain. Most forms of treatment have limitations.

Remember that:

- *Some drugs and medication have damaging side-effects.*
- *Surgery may relieve pain but it does not always give total relief or mobility.*
- *No treatment is going to restore lost youth!*
- *No one has discovered a magic formula to deal with all pain, whatever claims may be made.*
- *We shall be wasting our lives if we chase one new 'cure' after another.*

There are a number of practical ways in which we can help ourselves. Here are just three:

☐ **Check for simple adjustments that may lessen pain**
- Is the mattress right?
- Do I need one pillow less — or more?
- Should I lose weight?
- Do I need an eye test or a new set of dentures?
- Do my feet need some expert attention?
- Should I swallow my pride and wear flat shoes?

☐ **Check on posture**
- Am I at the right height when I type, sew, write or work in the kitchen?

- Do I stand and sit correctly?
- Do I move or sit awkwardly? When we are in pain, we tend to hold our bodies rigid in an attempt to protect painful areas. This is called 'muscle-guarding'. It actually makes matters worse, so try to correct awkward posture or movement.

☐ **Check on daily chores**
- When carrying, two even loads are better than one heavy one.
- Don't work too long against the pain. Do painful tasks in easy stages.

Monitoring the pain, over a short period, may help. Use a rating of one to five and note the level of pain at certain set times of the day. At the same time record what you are doing. This can help to show what triggers the pain as well as what diverts it. Now use the information to help keep pain levels low.

It's Not Just the Pain!

Putting up with pain is bad enough, but chronic pain may bring added, unwanted baggage.

• Tiredness

'It isn't just the pain,' Jenny complained, 'it's feeling so tired. I hardly know how to drag myself around sometimes.'

Chronic pain *does* make us tired, and when we're tired we are more likely to feel negative and unable to cope. So it's important to try to avoid reaching the stage of utter exhaustion.

It's tempting, on a good day, to do all the jobs that have been piling up, but that may mean getting so tired that you can't do much for the next few days.

Psychologists encourage us to break this kind of see-saw pattern and to build alternating periods of rest and activity into our daily schedule.

It's important to save our energy for the things that matter most.

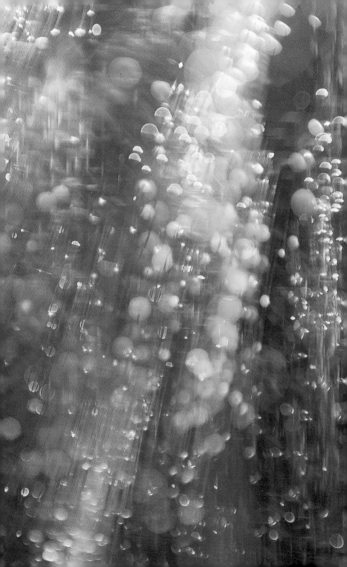

Molly was told that she must cut down on
a too-busy programme. She chose to resign from
a stressful committee that also involved a tiring
journey.

*Sometimes, a very special occasion can be worth the
pain and tiredness that will follow.*

Jane badly wanted to attend a reunion of past
colleagues and friends. She cut out other engage-
ments beforehand and made sure she had time to
recover afterwards.

- **Stress**

All kinds of circumstances — and people — make
us uptight. Stress affects our bodies as well as our
minds and makes the pain worse.

*It is important to look for ways to reduce stress, by
easing situations or relationships that cause it.*

But pain causes stress, as well as stress causing
pain. When pain is severe, our muscles tense up, just
as they do when we are nervous or anxious.

Most of us have our own way of reducing stress
— taking a warm bath, listening to music, or
whatever it may be. It is important, too, to learn
how to relax — at relaxation classes, or with help
from a doctor, or even from a book. Practise the
technique regularly, ready to use whenever the pain
is bad.

If you are keeping a daily record of pain levels,
add another column, headed stress. Put a score,
from one to five, rating your stress level, and
note against it what is happening, or what you are
thinking or feeling at the time. This helps to

pinpoint some causes of stress so that you can deal with them.

• Depression

We all feel a bit blue at times, but people coping with chronic pain may suffer from the kind of depression that needs medical treatment. Even when there is no accompanying depression a doctor may prescribe anti-depressants, because they can sometimes help to relieve chronic pain.

11

Distracting the Pain

We learn from experience that pain is worse at some times than at others. When we are enjoying ourselves with friends, or doing work we like, we don't notice the pain as much as when we lie awake at night.

Various factors determine how much we *feel* the pain.

Look at the lists in the box. There is a lot we can do for ourselves to keep the gate shut and the pain out.

Being with other people helps. Those who live or work alone need to find opportunities to mix socially and resist the temptation to become solitary and inward-looking.

There are many ways of keeping our minds busy. Here are just a few:

- books
- television and radio
- puzzles and mind-teasers

The Gate Control Theory

This pictures a gate to the brain which can open to let pain messages through, or shut to keep them out.

Some things that open the gate are:

- physical damage
- lack of activity — we notice pain more when we do less
- depression — feeling that we are helpless in our situation
- anger
- fear
- stress
- giving too much attention to the pain

Things that help to close the gate include:

- pain-killers
- massage, heat treatment or cold compresses
- keeping busy
- mental stimulus, meditation
- relaxation

- classes — on flower arrangement, archaeology, or anything that interests us
- at night, when we lie awake, we can plan a garden, a dinner menu, or a novel, with no worry about how much it will cost or the hard work involved.

Psychologists tell us that there are strict limits to what our conscious mind can hold at any one time. If we fill the front of the mind with interesting thoughts and ideas, we shall push the pain to the back, where we want it to be.

The Power of Positive Thinking

The person who is determined to get on top of the pain and who adopts a positive attitude, copes far better than the one who says, 'It's not fair! Why should this happen to me?'

Professor Martin Seligman, of the University of Pennsylvania, believes that what he describes as 'having a "yes" in your heart', makes for achievement and psychological health.

We may agree that it's the positive people who cope best with life, but that may not be much comfort. If you are not optimistic by nature, what can you do about it?

There *are* ways of dealing with unhelpful, negative responses:

- *Self-absorption* locks us into a little world of our own misery. Instead, practise thinking of others, and offer any help that you are able to give.
- *Grumbling* can become a bad habit. There are so

many things to be thankful for. Practise 'counting your blessings'.

- *Guilt* — real or imagined — can weigh you down. But there is no need to carry this burden.
  God offers us forgiveness in Jesus, who himself shouldered the consequences of our wrongdoing. Take up that offer.
- *Resentment and bitterness*, however justified, destroy us. When God forgives us, he also helps us to forgive others.
- *Fear* about what may happen tomorrow — or in ten years' time — makes us tense and anxious.
  God is the perfect parent. We can safely trust our future to him.

Being positive is not just a matter of temperament. We can train ourselves to react in positive ways.

Best of all, we can decide to put ourselves unreservedly into God's hands. When we trust him we can face life with genuine optimism. He promises to care for us and be with us whatever happens.

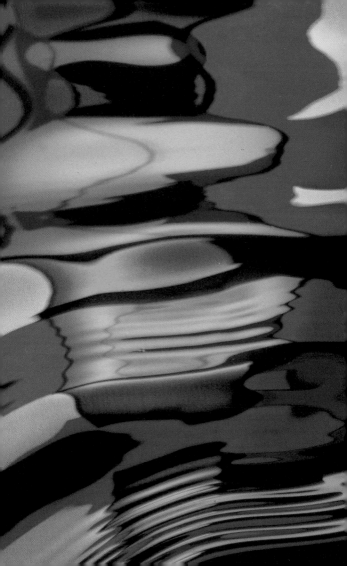

Relating to Others

'People like us don't belong anywhere. Those who are fit don't make allowances for us. We have to compete on equal terms or not at all. The seriously disabled don't accept us either. They envy us because we can still do so much that they can't.'

Caroline, who suffers from osteo-arthritis, describes how many of us feel. We need to learn how best to relate to those we work and live with.

Margery lives alone. She would love more people to come and see her. But only a few are ready to put up with the long, detailed account of aches and pains that she gives to everyone she meets.

It's usually best to say nothing, except to a close friend or a fellow sufferer.

When we don't *look* disabled, others may make unreasonable demands. It's good to tackle everything we can, but we must explain firmly when a task or activity is too much.

Pain makes us vulnerable, and we can easily be upset by others' reactions. It helps to try to see the funny side and learn to laugh at ourselves.

Asking for help poses problems, especially for those living alone.

Marian discovered: 'Certain relationships take only so much strain. People *say* they are willing to help, but, when you ask, they are afraid of long-term involvement.'

She has tried to adjust her way of living so that she cuts down on things she can't do herself. She recognizes that it is all right to ask for help, but not to impose. She saves her requests for the things that are really important.

Family life can be affected when one member is coping with chronic pain. Tact and thought are needed to keep relationships healthy.

Some use pain as a weapon against their nearest and dearest. In subtle ways, we can prevent those close to us from living their own lives, or make them feel guilty when they do.

Sometimes we become locked into a negative pattern of behaviour. Constant complaining can make a partner or close relative feel resentful, then guilty. The person in pain may also feel resentment at not being sufficiently considered. That can lead to guilt feelings too.

Love and mutual satisfaction cannot flourish when two people are caught in the complaint-resentment-guilt trap.

Loving relatives may mistakenly offer too much sympathy or help. It is important to go on doing as

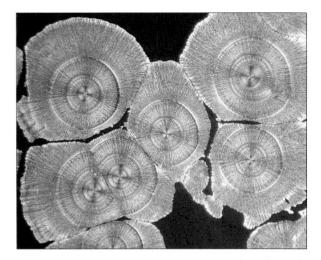

many jobs as you can, even if it takes twice as long.
Once you acquire the role of invalid it's hard to lose.
And that's bad for the whole family.

Common Responses

People who live with chronic pain respond in various ways, not all of them helpful.

Sometimes pain becomes a convenient excuse. By all means make sensible decisions in the light of your disability, but don't use pain as a substitute for the real reason behind your actions.

Pain keeps us on a short fuse. Extra effort is needed just to cope with everyday living. It is tempting, when life gets on top of us, to take it out on others. Unfortunately, we usually choose to snap at those who are below us in the pecking order. The children, or juniors in the office, shouldn't suffer because *I'm* in pain.

Self-pity is another pitfall to avoid. There will be days when you feel sorry for yourself. Learn to major on the good things you still enjoy, and to think of others, until it becomes a habit.

Projecting the blame for our condition on to other people does no good either. Sooner or later we must come to terms with our situation and take responsibility for how we live in the present.

Not all unconscious responses to pain are bad or negative. Dr Paul Tournier, a Swiss physician trained in psychiatry, found that those who achieve most in the world are often the ones who have been deprived in some way or another.

Loss of health can actually motivate us to achieve in other areas. We may develop hidden creative talents, or invest our energies in some worthwhile cause.

When we are aware of what is going on in our minds, we can foster helpful responses and refuse to let the negative ones take over.

15

A Purpose in Pain

Human beings need to find purpose in life. Some may accept the idea that life is meaningless and random, but most of us, recognizing the pattern that exists in nature, look for a pattern in our own lives too.

Is there any meaning in pain? Has it any purpose in my life?

In *The Problem of Pain*, C.S. Lewis wrote:

'Pain insists upon being attended to. God whispers to us in our pleasures . . . but shouts in our pains: it is his megaphone to a deaf world.'

God *does* want to speak to us but, when life is going smoothly, we often don't listen. Pain makes us stop and ask questions. Pain is never good, but God is able to take the worst things that happen to us and use them for our greatest benefit.

God is concerned with our lasting good. This life is only a fraction of our existence. God wants us to discover the true purpose for which we were made immortal, by finding him.

Pain turns our attention to these important questions of life. It may also bring us to the end of our own resources, and enable us to rely on God.

God wants us to hear his good news — that Jesus, for our sake, voluntarily took on pain. He died, but he rose to life again. Through Jesus, God:

- offers us forgiveness and a new quality of life
- shows us, by example, how to endure suffering
- assures us of his understanding and sympathy
- gives us his help and his company as we wrestle with pain.

Benjamin Franklin said: 'Those things that hurt, instruct.' Pain can play an important part in helping us to grow up and mature as human beings.

Our pain can help others too, because it can make us more sensitive and understanding. When we are in need of help and advice, we go to someone who has experienced suffering as well as success. Such people speak from the heart.

It could just be that pain is the best thing that's happened to us!

The Voice of Experience

'I sometimes think that to talk of "fighting pain",
when it's at its worst, is the wrong approach,'
Patricia says. 'It is necessary to go along with the
pain — to accept it.'

John's pain is the result of an industrial accident.
'When the pain is really bad,' he says, 'I'm too tired
and weak to do more than cling to one of God's
promises — verses like: "The eternal God is your
refuge and underneath are the everlasting arms."'

Kate actually visualizes her pain, and the accompanying
fears and anxieties, as a heavy pack. She
pictures herself taking it off her back, and handing it
over, piece by piece, to God.

David is a soccer enthusiast. When his pain is
at its sharpest, he fills his mind with images of the
game. He imagines that he is playing for the team he
supports, tackling, shooting, scoring goals.

Carlo Caretto has suffered a lifetime of pain. In *Why O Lord?* he shares his own 'little trick' for coping when the pain is at its worst:

- **Pray** a simple prayer, remembering that 'help comes to me from the Lord, who made heaven and earth'.

- **Find** some act of love to perform, in words or in action.

- **Wait:** for 'it is good to wait in silence for God to save'.

'Then I usually fall asleep,' he adds, 'so I don't know what happens next. But — at last — I feel better.'